Genetic Processing.

© Bradley William Strik.

Condition of Sale : The information contained within this book is intellectual property under copyright of the author and is only for the personal use or education and entertainment of the book purchaser. The material may not be used as part of operations of governments, corporations, charities, orders or religions but may only be used by a non religious not for profit's with costed supervision by the author personally.

© Bradley William Strik.

Dedication

This book is dedicated to Tim Strik. A man that kept one hand on the book of law and the other hand tinkering with machinery. With this Tim and Alex taught me scientific method.

© Bradley William Strik.

(Quote)
"A Science will come from Psychoanalysis that will ensure the Longevity of Man".
– Jung.

Introduction

This book is the initiator of a infant science born from an old science that deals with the harnessing of the three dimensional "screen" you see when you close your eyes. The Mind Space. In the new millennium human potential has taken steps towards stagnation. It is just so hard to get anything done. We blame government red tape, burgeoning corporations or overseas powers but in truth it is that we are coming to the end of an age. Prosperity of old forged by the rail magnates was the highlight of an age long gone that many try to replicate but present day "entrepreneurs" are only capable of mild economic improvements and medium sized project aspirations. Company secretaries of ocean trading companies wielding absolute power over the seas no longer act as the overseers that disseminate their will and haul shared riches back to their home ports. Those days are gone. Survival against the threat of nature and lawless barbarians or pirates is just not as much of an issue as it was before. But guard is still held as there are still items that come of these old ideas, the seed of which we are still hoping to remove. Things in general are less extreme. Greatness no longer propels an individual to the top it just raises them slightly above a few and lifts them in under a few others. Bravery and courage issue forth. Morality and philosophy meet them on the path and question them. They are a little confused with their rashness removed so bravery and

© Bradley William Strik.

courage are now maybe just, but importantly, a stable desire to help. These shifts point to the fundamental change that has taken place and that leads to a way up.

Parts of humanity have lifted the core underlying governing belief that guides their principle direction to Prosper.

Things that we once knew to be true we are being asked to question. These items are often still true in a sense or under specific conditions but not under all as assumed before. New sciences, methods and awarenesses will emerge from this fundamental shift for humanity. Part of this shift is that the small things are now important. Old ideas will now be discarded for a time or refreshed. There is a tiny infinitesimally small shift that has made it possible for a new scientific component of the science of old style psychoanalysis, genetics and memory that, I believe, has the potential to raise the genetic structure of individuals connected through the human genome to such a degree that the accomplishment of humanity is all fields of worthwhile endeavour will triple the total cumulative achievements humanity has made from the beginning of history in the next 30 years. For that I feel enthusiastic. I must now settle and curb my optimistic hopes so that I can pass without error, slanting or omission a technically perfect body of knowledge to the reader that will for the future be an antithesis of marketing but a helpful science – Genetic Processing.

© Bradley William Strik.

Chapter: Researched to the Breakpoint.

The teams of researchers stopped. They were looking around in wonder at each other proud of what they had just done but slightly remorseful because they would not need to come in tomorrow, or the next day or ever again. The reason being, they had tied a knot in every single loose end of the research without flaw and as a reward for years of hard work they must now walk out to look for new work never able to mention or talk about the discoveries they had made. What was different was that this was not another corporate success story that meant mass individual failure. No. In the afternoon as they filed out of the building and handed their security cards to the bald headed security guard whose head shone with the sweat that lathering it reflected in the light while each of the researchers and administrative support staff took with them a foundational scientific or administrative framework that had led to complete prosperity.

The chief executive officer stood side by side with her personal assistant just outside the front door handing out a small basket of gifts with an information pack filled to the brim with helpful information about finding a new career, what pitfalls to avoid in the search and where the best work opportunities were to be found. There was the tiny insignia of the private research firm alongside the logo of the human resources organisation that was contracted to put the information together for the valued staff. Research had reached a breakpoint.

The breakpoint was that all attempts to enhance the process led to the development of negative residuals or loss of efficiency or both.

© Bradley William Strik.

The research could go no further. There was no way to break the impasse but what was left was a completed science not a theory or suggested line of research rather a synthesised principle in action with no unresearched line of enquiry that humanity, once the principle in action was developed into a knowledge source – surrounded by all its supporting material, would be applied and mastered because of its completeness. And that is a remarkable achievement – Genetic Processing's Creation.

© Bradley William Strik.

Chapter : What does Genetic Processing Do.

Over the long term, possibly as long as twenty years, it should be theoretically possible for any illness to be cured with genetic processing but in the meantime while the genetic processor is diligently processing one would expect the severity of the illness to gradually lower as it is slowly withdrawn from the genome as happens under ideal circumstances while the patient is minimally treated medically to create the space so circumstances pressing in on the individual are not too grievous that then in process should make it possible to study the said cured or partially cured individual of both tissue and blood samples comparatively to the like from a healthy genetic processing processor so as to lead to medical advances in chemistry or approach making the enhancement of the physical body or curing of more illness a reality for applied medical science.

There are vast reservoirs of poverty associated memory stored in the beginning of the genome that can effectively be hereby removed in essence at the core instructional level with genetic processing where poverty is found growing in sufficient degree to inhibit the prosperity of an individuals non nerve memory source with sufficient ferocity as to keep poor the human race as there is unremoved fodder for at least two generations into the future on the genome which is in no way sorely missed by the processor that removes it or any of their family once removed to allow a natural level of prosperity to emerge on the "family memory source" or non nerve memory source.

A natural individual independent sense of morality of feeling naturally emerges from the practice of genetic processing such that complex structures of non nerve emotional pathways are

© Bradley William Strik.

established that enhance survival or prosperous natures of the body that further develop into the fabric of the body pathways that enhance it's path through life and uphold a sense of being right even when faced with massive adversity or pressure from other bodies such that a break is needed in status quo to alleviate general non nerve pressures set up by incorrect processes of thought that try to shut out our higher feelings.

In summary the health benefits, reduction of poverty and higher sense of moral feeling that come from genetic processing makes it a worthwhile process.

© Bradley William Strik.

SECTION : NO RELIGION.

(Quote)
"Titans help Humanity with their feeling. God's issue vengeance with their thoughts".
- Pythagorus.

Chapter : Destruction of the genome

"So what you are saying to me, young man, is that if I spill a few drops of paint into the lake when I am paining a Monet you will investigate; yet if I want to build a religious system of power that hurls using withheld genetic links on bilirubin in the bile of the body destructive magnetism or deabilitating radiation or high frequency waves into every passerby thus the human genome creating mass poverty and spread of human illness which will in the future be scientifically provable you will not do a single thing to stop, curtail or clean up this practice.
Hello. Hello. Hello."
The Genetic Processing CEO slowly lowers the phone, breathes out a short sharp breath, relaxes back into her chair and sighs.

The only two correct uses of the mind space are sleep and genetic processing.

The Genetic Processing CEO jumps from her chair, running a few short steps as is required in heels to be graceful and settles into a purposeful stride towards the double doors at the far side of the

© Bradley William Strik.

office. The three directors are present. "Morning company secretary", one of them greets her – a confident, humble man with a broad smile. A skinny man with his arms folded and squinting eyes gets straight to the topic of importance "What do you think of the intent of the corporate purchase offer for the firm". "Hmm", she gathers. "It places us in a position of having our technologies released slowly to a few demanding higher paying clients for a largish upfront fee while keeping from the as bread to butter benefactors technology that would be broadly helpful leading to a stable loyal market of end benefactors that will zealously expand for us the dispersal of this and later technological innovations to required humane bodies of knowledge in directions that we choose to apply our knowledge development nouse to in the future". All three directors raise their hands - "Proceed".

© Bradley William Strik.

Chapter : Twisted Memory.

Allowance of religious freedom for thousands of years has led to contortion of memory through religious practice to such an extent that there is memory in Mitochondria of the human body that is not in keeping with the optimum functioning of the body with both the Red Blood Cells and Non Nerve Cells containing this mitochondrial memory leading the human body away from the medical optimum for which it is capable which with the Genetic Processing lead puts the Human Body and potentially one day the Human Genome into an era where one day we may all be like the walking Titans of mythology with a prime optimum functioning body that Does Not weaken itself with mitochondria stored memory.

Religion is to blame but for them we feel no hatred.

The science of genetic processing fundamentally does not have any animosity towards religion as might be thought but rather it views religion like a child making a mistake for the way religion as a general but not sole culprit has twisted the DNA by experiencing euphoric states in the Mind Space. In general to place a perspective here, emotion removed, a religion is a structure like a government, company, charity, trust or not for profit with the unique purpose of a religion being to destroy something. e.g.

Catholicism was set to destroy Sin but eventually operated to remove Unpunished Crime.
Islam was set to destroy All that is not Islam but now operates to remove The non Utopia.
Hinduism set itself to destroy Money to replace it with caste but

© Bradley William Strik.

now undermines Greed.
Buddhism was founded to destroy Evil but is now an instrument to remove War.

In the destruction the practices of these organisations lift up their members by twisting their DNA causing damage to themselves and others. Predominantly in the form of Poverty or Sickness. Those that do Genetic Processing sometimes have difficulty wading through the damage caused by the twisting of the religious practitioners DNA to make the religious practitioner relatively more powerful as the processor is only lifting the DNA to create improvement not Twisting and lifting. It is good for the processor to remember that in cleaning up the mess of the twisting it is in truth their work that has moved humanity towards a lawful utopia free of war and greed.

© Bradley William Strik.

Chapter : System of Power or System of Emancipation

It is important to understand that there is a difference between a system of emancipation which allows you to stand with others supporting them and a system of power, traditionally religious methods, that allow you to stand above others outside of the religious structure to gain advantage over them that from the human interaction view places Genetic Processing as a true system of interactive human emancipation where the processor is not superior to others in spirit because of their application of Genetic Processing leading them away from wanting to cause a genetic conflict that will lead a religious system of power to potentially unwind as it completely lowers the position of a religious body from existence should it's members engage in the Genetic Processing process or it's organising body should endorse the use of genetic processing but there will be an additional avoidable processing penalty that forms on the DNA of a processor seeking to intentionally cause harm to religions, religious bodies or religious persons in such a way that the natural inclination for a genetic processing processor is to work on more productive endeavours away from religion preferring religious avoidance.

Genetic Processing applied by religions, religious bodies or religious persons will scientifically undermine their system of power or religion and lead to it's decline or potential removal.

© Bradley William Strik.

SECTION : TITAN.

(Quote)

Strong, masterful and capable in all areas of life.
Above the Gods and Goddesses on occasion.
Preferring the non religious as their companions.
Fearing the retribution of Gods when below Them.
– Zeus.

Chapter : TITAN of Powerful Feeling.

Titan is the optimum outcome state of Genetic Processing which is both masculate* and feminine. *masculate : to man as feminine is to woman. Incorrectly worded masculine in the past.

Bound for family glory in the highest degree and in all possible ways demonstrating physical strength based on optimum genetic body structure based on their race with the optimum IQ for their travels through this life guided by powerful accurate feelings as they prosper in life guided by a sense of personal virtue written up in creed, moral code or doctrine as a physical antithesis of mental illness they raise the spirit of humanity by lifting with gradual improvement their DNA along with that of those around them whilst also being great friends to have with an inclination away from religion demonstrating proficiency in profession or the arts far and above the lowly stated normal for which we have been told to be content that will be no more be with the rise of the titans.

© Bradley William Strik.

Levels of Feeling
Glory
Joy
Happy
Content
Neutral

Measure of feeling for a Titan starts at neutral lifts to content, then on to happy with joyful above topped by Glory sought at ever rising levels at the peak.

The Titan is guided by higher feeling not emotion as the definition of emotion has shifted in the language to suggest some type of expression that is weak or needy where the strength of feeling that guides the titan with optimism uplifts those around them as they become a presence that raises the environment they are in while maintaining a quite control acting outside the guidance of the gods at times then at other times under Their pressure but all the time open hearted remembering to assist not hinder as a friend to man while they await the next opportunity to rise to glory that they may realise higher levels of realisation for themselves and their human ties.

Chapter : Virtues for a Titan.

The Genetic Processing CEO takes her high-heels off spreads her arms out like a T and collapses back into the lounge at home to the onomatopoeia of "push". There is the shout of her child. "Here comes the titan", he says. Jennifer catched her child as he flies through the air straight at her and gently places him on the lounge next to her. "Did you slave for those gods all day religious

© Bradley William Strik.

woman", he continues in play. "The directors", Jen shortly enquires, "It was harrowing". "Did you learn the secrets held by the gods about the titans, my spy?" the child questions further. Jennifer pauses for a while – then wings it.
"I will tell you the virtues of a titan …."

1. Always be Sensible.
2. Do not do things to regret.
3. No smoking.
4. No violence.
5. No Alcohol.
6. Have HUMILITY.

"A Titan hates to talk about weakness my son. So for all titans or budding titans it will be short. Glory thurst may take away your sensability. Do not let it.
When 'beneath the gods' you fall into emotion some times. Do not wreck-havoc or apply violence. Instead rest till settled if disturbed, unsettled or in discontent.
Human vices like drugs, smoking and alcohol will drop you from titan to human. Allow it not.
Do what is required to have a good relationship with your spouse. Love your spouse. Adore you children. Respect your parents. Family matters.
If you exercise humility when you feel strong you may not experience weakness when 'the gods are above you'. I say that in inverted commas because there are no gods left as the titans have taken over".
So if you don't have humility and use manners in this home a mommy will tickle you thinks Jen. "Ah He Ha Ha Ha" she says as she tickles the boy.

© Bradley William Strik.

SECTION : WHAT IS THE MINDSPACE?

The MindSpace is the world that exists when you close your eyes that takes us to our dreams, if used correctly, or to our demise - if not.
- Test Subject One.

Chapter : Jung, Creator or Explorer.

Jung was the most notable in the field of psychoanalysis not psychiatry that opened or found the MindSpace with his ideas on the collective unconscious - a glimpse at the factual existence of the interaction of the various human DNA on the human genome and the human genome itself which became something that in his time even the most advanced understandings of the the science of psychoanalysis was not able to be accurately establish as a scientific tenet as it is now used in the science of Genetic Processing.

Jung was the first opener and explorer of the MindSpace.

Jung's use of the MindSpace stands above all others in history as it opens up the possibility of alleviation of pressure on the mentally ill in contradiction to religious MindSpace uses that position the mentally afflicted as those being of raucous demon possessed nature that are on their way to one of the myriad hells of mind or location to be controlled and submitted to barbarism that historically may have meant treatment in torture chambers

© Bradley William Strik.

which would leave the mentally afflicted further down trodden with none to help as they are thus segregated outside the bounds of those worthy of compassion, the excluded, that they be held away from upliftment by spiritual distortion in the MindSpace that in any event would not improve them or minimise their symptoms.

© Bradley William Strik.

Chapter : Born From Psychanalysis.

Typically psychoanalysis is a practice where the analyst helps a patient to in the comfort of their well reclined couch go through memories coming to re-conclusions about past events of their life so as to create for the patient better bases for their life such that the patient achieves better outcomes and are better equipped to deal with life which developed into a practice of self psychoanalysis which is a little dangerous where the process is performed without the analyst in a kind of a poor man's psychoanalysis that has a set course where what happens though analysis is the individual involved moves through past memories in which re-conclusion becomes less important or happens naturally such that a pattern of particular types of memories are experienced and the grand discovery is that it is only memories with links to biliruben in the body that need to be experienced to improve the self-psychoanalyst and the self-psychoanalyst's path.

It is key to experience memories with eyes closed containing biliruben to benefit the brain, body and their future.

A safe method to do so is explained at the end of the book so that you need not experience the tribulations and inturbulations that others travelling the road before you have gone through in order to produce the said safe method extracted from the basement of self-psychoanalytic practice so that many of us may benefit from a honed high functioning brain directed body that is not limited by the medium sized aspirations of a human past forming from a practice that can be widely applied while easily understood to take the part of humanity involved in the takeup of Genetic Processing to the level of humanity to which they choose to rest.

© Bradley William Strik.

Chapter : You're going to Priam.

This chapter is about reframing of damage on front of DNA in the MindSpace because of an old idea taking form there that may cause a person after processing to feel, hopefully falsely, that they are going to prison which needs be immediately dealt with in the exercise of a self reframing from the negative "You are going to prison" to 'You are going to Priam' who was the king at the height of Troys prosperity or perhaps a younger living one you know because there is a great deal of prosperity in the memories of the time leading up to the violent greek poetry with a large slump of the memories of downfall giving cause to such a reframing as the ideal way to deal with this side effect that sometimes comes from the processing that is not of the processing.

© Bradley William Strik.

SECTION : MEMORY AND YOUR PART OF THE MINDSPACE.

Chapter : The 3 memory sources of your body.

There are 3 memory sources in the human body. They are:-
Red Blood Cell Memory Source.
Non Nerve Cell Memory Source.
Nerve Cell Memory Source.

Mitochondrial memory in the red blood cells and non nerve cells are an error of memory discussed in an earlier chapter as it applies to the human body. Mitochondrial memories if still present in the different cells of a human share commonalities but also have differences in the different cells but are returned to more accurate locations and gradually disappear from the erroneous locations with the application of Genetic Processing.

Likewise, nerve memory and non nerve memory also share commonalities but they are essentially different memory sources containing different memories. Non nerve cells hold genetic memory of feeling in their nucleus and sometimes the mitochondrial memory outside their nucleus. Nerve cells have genetic memory of thought in their nucleus with not the erroneous mitochondrial memories outside it. Red blood cells will generally, at the time of writing, have only mitochondrial memory with no genetic memory of their own until such time as there is no mitochondrial memory in the cells of the body and the body appropriately reconfigures itself. All three memory sources are inter reliant whereby subtle changes created in one lead to subtle

© Bradley William Strik.

changes in another with platelets sometimes appearing to have a mitochondria where in fact they merely grabbed hold of a mitochondria to remove something undesirable but also beneficial changes are prevented in one memory source on the basis that such changes will lead to detrimental change in a different memory source.

Effecting change in memory to bring about improvement is gradual.

The non nerve memory source stores memories of feeling passed to the individual from their ancestry and a notable radical in genetic processing has suggested the current and past lives of a person are found in the nerve memory source in thought based memories of the human being.

The genetic memories as stored in the non nerve memory source are more to do with feeling while the memories stored in the nerve memory source are related to thought.

Correctly held together the interactive drive of the cumulative memory line, at optimum, of the human being is for the forward most red blood cell memory to pull in the non nerve memory behind followed by the nerve memory.

© Bradley William Strik.

Chapter : Aspects.

If we can imagine the brain for the moment to be like a computer with Windows running are like the MindSpace with different windows open representing different aspects of the mindspace which relate to different aspects of life, some of these aspects as they appear at first are negative, but later on they form up as all positive as listed below with each aspect forming a very specific role in leading the body with incentive to greater prosperity such that a complete prosperity with little chance of reversal is set at a stable incline for the brain and body to follow and improve.

At the Survive Level the aspects are as follows :-
Army
Heaven
Sanity
Sexuality
Waste
Sex
Crime Removal
Happiness
God
Human needs
Work
Earth
Law
Operate
Family
Riches
Psychiatry
Titan
Neck

© Bradley William Strik.

Armour
Death

Documents

With a natural balanced attention to the different aspects at times appropriate the body and the life that it leads will be balanced positively.

© Bradley William Strik.

Chapter : Brief; The full gambit of memory.

-Memory
-DNA
-Genome

The Genetic Processing CEO, Jennifer, floats into the the boardroom on her new high heels for the latest brief on the MindSpace certain that the work that is going on is about to reveal more about the existance of memory links between people in the same families then more broadly to races and on to humanity as a whole as the scientist in the starched white lab-coat takes the floor in front of the digital display board where slide upon slide is put up to confirm the thoughts of Jennifer on the subject with links between memory, DNA and the Genome the conclusion of the research that had painstakingly with great attention to detail put in place to further understand the extent to which the MindSpace affected human lives on all levels. Jennifer is happy with the progress.

From small scale to large scale memory has links on the levels of individual, DNA and the genome.

Individual memory secures identity marking the space where the personal contribution is formed which integrates with the collective memory of family which is dominant on the DNA that shows itself able to, incredibly slowly, in a very controlled way be altered in the Genetic Processing process with on to the larger view of memory the personal memory sits inside the DNA which itself sits inside the Genome - the entirety of recollected memory of the human race. The genome has been incorrectly labelled by Psychoanalysis when first found in the Mind Space as the collective unconsciousness.

© Bradley William Strik.

SECTION : LEANING ON PSYCHIATRY.

Chapter : Curing mental illness.

First Quarter.
Jennifer picked up Eric by his shirt held tightly around his throat and said "You are just not trying hard enough to cure your mental illness". Just then a scientist walked in with two large cups of coffee. "Put him down Jen", he said continuing "I have it figured out". "I do not want coffee at a time like this" commented Jennifer - "I do not think he is trying hard enough". The scientist cooled the situation with "He cannot access the memories clearly because of his psychiatric meds but 4 shots of coffee should perk him up and give him clarity of mind to access memory without stopping his meds. "Drink up Eric" said the scientist as he handed eric the two cups of coffee.

Second Quarter.
The scientist reported "we sorted out the inability to clearly access memory last quarter with the four shots of coffee for people on psychiatric meds, today the difficulty for Eric appears to be that the MindSpace breaks a mental illness up into many parts and when part of the mental illness collapses out of the mind space another lesser part rises up stronger than before". "So what is Eric doing" asked Jennifer. "Sticking to the basics and riding it through" said the scientist.

"How are you feeling?" asked Jennifer. Eric replied "This is the only hope to cure my mental illness so I am working through it. Thanks for the opportunity".

© Bradley William Strik.

Chapter : Electric Shock Treatment, Questioning a False Tenet.

Third Quarter.
Jen is watching a video of a scientist interviewing Eric. "Well I went back to my Psychiatrist and had my meds adjusted for the changes to my psychiatric condition. There was a small hospital admission involved but I needed to settle back down. At least I know that with the processing I am not as bad as the other patients who have to go in for electric shock treatment and the like. They come out horrible and look to be the tormented of an already tormented body" Jen stops the tape.

Fourth Quarter.
Jennifers fists clench in a controlled rage as she shuffles through the reports on her desk numerous in number confirming that shock treatment working is a false scientific tenet perpetuated by it's patients in research saying they feel better in order to avoid further treatment which creates great anguish in her brain because as a scientist she knows the practice will continue to harm people until such a time as the scientific community as a whole gather against the False Tenet in an established science and take it from practice but in the mean time her heart bleeds for those that must suffer.

© Bradley William Strik.

SECTION : PRESSURE ALLEVIATION.

Sometimes pressure will build up in a person after processing and below are six things you can do to alleviate that pressure :-

Location Shift

Location Shifting is moving around to different sub-locations to create personal stability.

If you are having a restful day at home try out the different locations around the place. Don't just veg out on your favourite lounge chair in front of the television. Read a book in a quite alcove. Let go in the garden. Afternoon nap in the bedroom. Rest for a while in the kitchen or dining area. Wait till a particular location becomes no longer personally endorsing before moving on to another location. Do not stagnate in a single location spread yourself over the different areas of operation in your locality to keep each location fresh. Try it at home then extend it to other environments where practical.

Recount with others period of happiness.

Recounting with others periods of happiness or happy stories or funny stories is a great way to settle yourself in order to get back into activity. The more the merrier.

Optimism

Looking to the best possible outcomes in the different events and activities going on around you is another great way to settle yourself into your activities.

© Bradley William Strik.

Close your eyes.

Sometimes the simplest things are the easiest. If pressure builds up from the processing just take some time to lay down and close your eyes without a processing instruction. Open your eyes momentarily if you go into a fall.

Eye Dancing

After you finish processing let you eyes dance around the different objects and different room components in the room where you are processing. Eye dancing helps to restore stability. The eyes move toward something then settle on it. It is not the eyes roughly barging on to everything that can be seen – It is Eye Dancing.

Take a Walk

Sometimes just simply taking a walk will allow the pressure to settle.

© Bradley William Strik.

SECTION : THE 16 AXIOMS.

The 16 Axioms are the assumptions and rules of the processing that are there to guide and rule it's application

*1.5m : When processing you need to remain at least 1.5m from another person. So you do not do it when sleeping next to another person. In exceptional circumstances where people are living in bunked arrangements it can be brought down to 0.8m but is best kept at the 1.5m
*FACT1:You ; The processing is about you and must always come back to you. Often it will take you far from your own memory sources so that you may feel you are not yourself but it must always come back to you. Never forget who and what you are.
*Lay Flat : The processing is done laying flat on your back.
*Must be Safe : The processing is designed to be safe or given rules to make it safe.
*Must cure mental illness : A basic principle of the processing is that it begin and remain an instrument to cure mental illness.
*Must work reliably : The processing is consistent in it's application and will continue to perform its duty to those using it.
*No electric light on : When processing do so without the electric light or lights in the room on. If you leave them on the processing will be adversely affected.
*No religion : To use Genetic Processing you need to not be religious as if you are religious it will not work.
*Prosperity interest : Using the processing brings forth ideas of prosperity and associated topics. It is suggested that if you are not into prosperity or will react negatively to prosperity then there will be a lot of struggle with no result.
* Science of MindSpace :The intent was that this volume was to

© Bradley William Strik.

initiate the removal of myth and misunderstanding from discussion and knowledge on the topic such that a science with stable accurate tenets be formed.

*Stop if disturbed by loud noises : One of the reasons where it is recommended that you take a break in processing. e.g. Emergency sirens, overly loud music etc. Just put it off to a time where there are no noise interruptions.

*Stop if disturbed : If someone comes in to the room or the phone rings. Take a break. Also do not process when others are on the phone.

*Stop if laugh : If you laugh or giggle when processing stop and restart or finish up.

*Stop if yawn, swallow or cough : If you do any of these three stop and restart or finish up.

*Take time to settle before and after processing : Not always possible but it is best if you take a moment to settle outside the MindSpace before and after.

*THE BIG RISK; Do not process into a fall.

THE MOST IMPORTANT AXIOM! If you are processing and you feel yourself falling or declining – STOP Processing- Then take a break.

© Bradley William Strik.

SECTION : THE FIRST SIX TENETS.

A Science is formed with tenets. As discoveries are made facts highlight themselves and hold up the other facts. The base six tenets or facts of Genetic Processing are as follows.

1. Genetic Processing Creates Prosperity : It removes poverty and creates prosperity, FACT.
2. Prosper : With continued use you will one day prosper, FACT.

Chapter : The 3 levels of being.

-Prosper.
-Survive.
-Perish.

Jennifer took up her seat to read through the latest reports of the floor testing of Genetic Processing that seemed to show that people from all walks of life were existing in the same spaces together but held into three very different angles depending upon their quality of memory such that beings in the middle were content to mosey along at a level of survive as different to those struggling to get by as they existed at a level of perish while up the top living like gods were those that found themselves lucky enough to have reached the level of being known as prosper.

© Bradley William Strik.

The level of being is lifted with the application of Genetic Processing.

3. Genetic Processing provides medical benefit. FACT.
4. Cures Mental Illness. Even the most complex of mental illnai are gradually disassembled, reduced and removed through the course of processing. FACT
5. Genetic Processing is a science that evolved from Psychoanalysis. Jungs entry into the MindSpace and the finding of the "collective unconsciousness" initiated an important series of events that allowed the emergence of Genetic Processing. FACT.

© Bradley William Strik.

Chapter : Tenet 6, Temper.

In the J.P. Getty book called How to Be Rich there is an item of discussion where it mentions that he has quit smoking but he is not against smoking. I read the book and as an editor author from an editing perspective thought it should be changed for a reprint to say that he was against smoking. But I erred in that I was not fully researched. The section of prose in question was worded to stop war. How? Smoking has not always been demeaned as solely cancer causing. Smoking used to be used by people to temper their thoughts to strengthen their outcomes. So when Getty was standing in his home America in the present day he would mentally declare himself to have more cash than the foreign debt, temper it down to him being the wealthiest merchant banker in the world then temper it down to him being the wealthiest merchant in his home country.

See, all can now be done without smoking.

Now say a General contemplating war was to puff on a cigarette saying "For What they did we will take them to war and slaughter every one of them". Wait a while. Another puff on a cigarette, "Maybe We can get a CeaseFire or a truce". More smoking. "Ah, it's not worth It".
N.B. As an ex-smoker I am personally against smoking.
*Temper : To bring down in intensity.

© Bradley William Strik.

SECTION : HARNESSING THE MINDSPACE.

Chapter : Why is Bilirubin so Special?

Bilirubin is memory waste that we believe to come from collapsed red blood cells. So in science to date the chemical is remarkably unspectacular. To Genetic Processing it serves as a guide leading the processor on a clearly marked and intricate path to genetic improvement. The memory which is current or as close to current as possible containing bilirubin is the most crucial memory that needs be experienced or re-experienced to raise the individual personally, in their family, in the DNA and on the genome. It is the yellow brick road of Genetic Processing – so when you start the process let it be the one and not the mind that leads you on a journey of self improvement. I warn you now. Sometimes things will not be pleasant.

If anything too difficult arises all you need do is open your eyes and it will stop.

© Bradley William Strik.

Chapter : Genetic Processing.

The process of Genetic Processing is simply a matter of reading a short phrase out before you close your eyes to initiate a sequence to bring about the outcomes achievable through Genetic Processing. In the phrase the last word of the phrase is repeated at the beginning to lock in the phrase and prevent the instruction being processed off by the process itself. It is also read without blinking or winking to keep continuity and isolation to the phrase. To blink or wink during reading the phrase out aloud is an error and doing so requires you close your eyes before opening your eyes and starting again. The phrase is spoken as it is read as the spoken word remains long after the thought word relinquishes it's control on the mind space. With that introduction the instructional line and the most powerful phrase in the world to improve the genome while being the core process of Genetic Processing is:-

Read the following out aloud with eyes kept open before closing eyes.

"bilirubin.
When I close my eyes now I must experience my current memory containing bilirubin."

You can try it for a short time now, perhaps five or ten minutes to start. Remember the Golden Rule and do not process into a fall. Be sure to use the ideas and understandings throughout the rest of the book that enhance it's value.

© Bradley William Strik.

Chapter : Non Fixation Treatment of Good Ideas

Good ideas sometimes arise when you are in the MindSpace. If the idea is truly great it will still be there for you after you finish processing. Sometimes there will be a sense of the ideas being lifted up to make them stronger and other times they just spring up before going away, either way do not let these ideas cause you to stop processing to write them down or grab hold of the idea with your concentration which will deter the processing.

Chapter : Uncomfortable Day Dreaming

Sometimes after a period after processing, sometimes the next day, a person will have a sensation of uncomfortable day dreaming. This happens because a person moves, usually as a means of protecting a person from future reversion potentially in any area of their life, off their own memory source. It is uncomfortable but when you take into account the other perspective on a different hand that you would have to go through unpleasant life experience if you did not move away from your memory source then it becomes acceptable.

© Bradley William Strik.

SECTION : Release.

Chapter : Revitalisation.

If you find the bilirubin processing line not to be working, a kind of build up of pressure because of the same or are having any other problems not covered in this written work then it probably means that there are adjustments being made to earlier memories that need to be settled down. It is done with a similar phrase to the bilirubin phrase used in the same manner as follows:

Read the following out aloud with eyes kept open before closing eyes.

"and magnetism.
When I close my eyes now I must experience my earliest memory containing radiation, magnetism or both radiation and magnetism."

Make sure you read the words as it uses "earliest" instead of "current" – not assuming both phrases are generally the same. Again if you feel a falling or declining sensation stop – by just opening your eyes and if you come across anything you have trouble dealing with just stop the process by just opening your eyes.

© Bradley William Strik.

Chapter : Set Sail.

Jennifer flicked through the small mini-book that she had taken from the crate ready to be be shipped for distribution. It was small. Concise. Accurate. Technically perfect in every detail. It had the answer to some of the problems of the world that people were battling with no real explanations that would help to overcome these problems. It would make a small mark to lighten the load of the downtrodden. Jennifer returned the small mini-book to the pallet of books as the forklift arrived.

© Bradley William Strik.

www.ingramcontent.com/pod-product-compliance
Lightning Source LLC
Chambersburg PA
CBHW031505210526
45463CB00003B/1085